Fighting Disease with Whole Food Nutrition

My Journey Fighting HIV with Whole Food Nutrition, Herbs and Spices

S. Diane Barry

Fighting Disease with Whole Food Nutrition

Copyright © 2017 by S. Diane Barry

ISBN 978-1546953500

Table of Contents

A Note from the Author

This book is my truth. It owes its concept to all the herbal remedies and alternative therapies thousands of years in the making.

You'll see "read about it" often because the books about herbs and natural therapies have already been written; just not about a real HIV fight with no meds, and no gimmicks.

I was scared when I was diagnosed. But I am doing ok, so far…and that's the best we can get.

I'll continue my path until it seems to not work any longer.

~S. Diane Barry

Dedicated To

All those who can't get "Meds" and to those who are afraid and think HIV is a death sentence.

To the Doctors who wish they could help their patients! And the people who have no health care.

This is about so much more than HIV.

It's about treating yourself like you want to be alive before you get a 'diagnosis'.

Don't wait and don't give up...you might be able to save your own life and the life of someone you love.

Introduction

I am writing this to inspire you to read more about HIV, or a condition you suffer from, to take part in your health and stop expecting doctors to work miracles.

As I come up on my 10th anniversary of my HIV positive diagnosis my body is hanging in there. I have seen correlations in lab results and life choices; including alcohol, cannabis, stress, kerosene fumes, exercise and an attack by wasps. My viral load reached 20,000 after the confrontation with a wasp nest, and soon after my body brought it back down in the 1000's range. No Meds!

When I began using Basil Oil, my VL went lower than any time since diagnosis with a 290 VL.

Everything you do can impact your health from spraying pesticides around your home to applying petroleum-based lotions on your skin. The fumes from plastic products, the chemicals in new carpet, and the stuff sprayed on your lawn, all accumulate in your body -especially in the winter when windows are closed and fresh air at a minimum.

You can eat microwaved convenience foods and pay for it later, or eat fresh fruits and vegetables, and reap the benefits, now and later.

Your Doctor isn't going to push the issue you, after all, have *free will*! And he makes money off your bad choices.

If you think might have HIV, **GET TESTED.** Testing early will give you the chance to make lifestyle changes that improve your bodies fight against the virus.

I REPEAT- testing early will give you the chance to make lifestyle changes, which will improve your body's fight against the virus.

This includes the fight against Hepatitis, STD's, and pre-cancerous conditions, and so many other conditions, diseases and ailments prevalent in today's *take a pill* mindset.

Prevention is easier than a cure.

Don't wait to get tested for HIV, waiting will waste precious time, possibly infect others, and could ruin your life...get tested and know your status!

I am not a Doctor. I am not a trained dietician. I am simply a *Whole Foods Enthusiast*!

I can't tell you what to do. You must decide to take better care of yourself for your own sake; no one can choose that for you. I did begin to study Health and Wellness, thinking that a Bachelor's Degree might serve me well but can tell you what I am doing without a degree. I make no claims of a cure or promises of anything. I only know what I am doing is working for me...so far...and I will admit when I am wrong or things change.

I have studied health and alternative therapies since I was young. My first encounter with alternative medicine happened in the 60's I was about 8 or 9. A young child was burned badly from a gasoline explosion and he was sent home to die. He came to my grandparents' house, along with a Healer. I was witness to herbal treatments and the healing of

this badly burned child.   It stuck with me. I realized that
doctors are not gods nor do they have all the answers.

My HIV Story

Let's fast forward to January 2005 when I got my HIV diagnosis. I have no idea when I actually was exposed. I have a pretty good idea- my Viral Load was low, in the 800's, when I was first diagnosed. I contracted it via sexual contact. Heterosexual contact and have no blame or harbor any bad feelings to who infected me. Thinking like that can only cause stress and feelings of guilt; neither is good for health and wellbeing.

One day, soon after my diagnosis, on World Aids Day, I heard a speaker from Africa say "Send us food! My people are not strong enough for the medicines; we need food to grow stronger!"

I thought to myself, "exactly!"

When I was diagnosed I never ran out and self-medicated. There was no binge drinking, no self-destructive behaviors. Many people get diagnosed and do things that make the situation even worse. I have never been a user of much of anything except Marijuana. I was never a coke head, a meth user, or a fan of alcohol. I hadn't damaged my immune system (Lymphatic system). I was always into health foods and healthy lifestyle choices, which probably served me well and placed me far ahead of others who may have damaged their healing capacity with drugs and alcohol.

This shows how important it is to eat healthily and avoid environmental toxins! You would think our health care professionals would advocate this, and maybe some do, but mine did not. They were often disengaged and distant with me. I am not on meds and do not need the medications. The doctors seem to be ill-equipped to relate to me. I ask questions they cannot answer. They do not seem interested in learning what I am doing or researching on my own.

I came across the Zephyr Foundation, a group for Elite Controllers and Non-Progressors, a virtually unknown group and a set of terms. I found few people who had ever heard of such a thing! With the help of my Primary Care Physician, my blood was submitted to Harvard Medical Center. I was not one of the lucky ones, yet here I am not on meds and not progressing. It is believed the Elite Controllers possess a gene from the Plague survivors that increases their disease resistance. I am of European decent, French even, but apparently my health is due to something else.

Diet and healthy lifestyle choices can only be the answer. Still, the medical community couldn't care less. I have tried to make noise, stir minds, raise awareness, and all of my efforts fall on deaf ears unwilling to hear what may be possible.

My most recent doctor's appointment was just another letdown, a waste of my time, and probably an insult to my healthcare professionals. They don't like to be contradicted, challenged, or disagreed with.

If you can't keep learning, you shouldn't be a doctor. You see, I told them I didn't want to be on meds – ever. That seemed to insult them. How dare a non-medical professional disagree with them? They totally bypassed the fact I was HIV positive but my viral load was only 290 – and I was on no meds.

In January 2013 my viral load was 290 and my CD4's were at 345. Three months later my viral load was 1209 and my CD4's at 456. I had hoped for an undetectable or lower number than the 290 from January, but I was reminded of my exposure to Kerosene fumes for about 5 days during the end of February, and I think it may have spiked the activity in my Viral Load, giving me the higher VL in April.

Most will focus on the low CD4's but I see them come right back up to battle the VL. Some folks have CD4's in the thousands, but I think that reflects a higher level of fighting going on. Of course, I am only guessing. It's a conversation healthcare professionals won't have with me. Their only answer is medication. I am not asking that question or willing to go their route. They have no answers for my questions so the conversation is over. I am left to do my own research.

So how did I get my viral load down to 290 without the meds? You would think the doctors would ask that question.

I am very angry with them that they do not ask, that they don't care enough or have enough curiosity to even inquire. Maybe I could have something of value to help others. I think I do. I am sorry doctors are so brainwashed, so closed minded, and so afraid to think outside the established medical community box.

I think a healthy foundation helps, but even if you have abused your body you can decide to make up for lost time. Work hard and give up alcohol and drugs. Don't go out and binge in despair and depression. It is time to make healthy choices and stick with it. It is time to read and research about HIV and what it does to you. Learn about the immune system and the lymphatic system.

Read about the herbs and spices recommended to fight viruses. Learn about the food additives and environmental toxins that are dangerous to your health. Take charge of your body and its care. I think there are more people out there doing the same as I am, but because no one wants to listen, they have stopped talking.

I was on a Facebook HIV group page, and a comment was made about coconut oil being a "cure". The majority of chatters were ready to lynch the commentator; he was attacked verbally and banned from the group.

Coconut oil contains lauric acid and is supposedly capable of eating the HIV virus. Whether it does or does not eat the virus it is extremely healthy for you. It is a welcome addition to your diet and a great part of a healthy lifestyle. Maybe you'd have to eat a pint of it a day to affect the virus, I don't know. But I did buy some. I do not use a pint of it a day but I use it. It makes excellent popcorn and fried potatoes, it works well with pancakes, and it makes a great body moisturizer and lubricant. I can only hope it also fights HIV even if only slightly. At least it makes you healthier and that will help fight the virus. I highly recommend that you read more about the benefits of coconut oil.

If every time someone comes up with an alternative therapy, someone else shoots the messenger, where will that get us? The messengers will stop talking, and I think that's where we are at. I do my own research. I read about herbs and spices, which ones kill bacteria and viruses. I obtained a medical book and learned the "immune system" is an intangible thing. It is the *lymphatic system* that is the nuts and bolts of our health.

Immune System/Lymphatic System = Mind/Brain. It is a good analogy. In learning how to heal and strengthen my immune system, I learned it was my lymphatic system that was the focus. Why in the hell don't health care professionals tell us this monumental bit of information?

They preach about strengthening the immune system, and it's basically misinformation. If you concentrate on the health and wellbeing of the lymphatic system you will be strengthening your immune system. Run that past your doctor.

So, back to my 290 viral load. After 8 years of extremely healthy eating, I have several theories about what may have brought it down, just as I have a theory about kerosene fumes bringing my viral load back up.

I had been using basil oil. Not every day, but often. Why? I have read that Basil and Oregano are anti-viral. Anti-Viral! I like the sound of that. I can't recommend that people taking pharmaceuticals try basil or oregano oil- maybe try eating more the herbs fresh. I will be continuing to use it and I hope that without the kerosene fumes, I'll see my viral load drop again.

Whole Food Nutrition

There are many alternative therapies. I believe that food is the best medicine. Nothing outrageous but a healthy diet of fresh foods, full of nutrition, is a good start.

Herbs and spices offer medicinal qualities that science seeks to replicate and reproduce. I believe in Mother Nature and choose the most natural options I can afford. Many will argue about the cost of health foods, but I will argue about the cost of health care -a cost I do not have! I often have to remind myself I am HIV positive. I am undoubtedly healthier than most of the people I know. I take no prescription medications other than an occasional muscle relaxer for neck pain. I even rely on a capsaicin or cayenne rub for topical use instead of taking a pill. I only use the medication as a last resort.

Prevention vs. cure is an excellent battle plan if you're serious about living healthy.

There are many other things that may contribute to my body holding this virus at bay. I am not a cigarette smoker. I am a Vegetarian. I never was a clean freak, so I don't use noxious chemicals to clean and pesticides are not my style.

Ants in the house? Put a saucer of sugar outside. Flies? Use fly tape. Wasps? A fake wasp nest will chase them (scare them) away. Fleas? Salt works well, it kills them. I am not a fan of flea collars, chemicals are BAD. And we use far too many of them!

And we eat far too many of them.

Speaking of salt- there are claims of table salt causing inflammation and swelling thus the Sea Salt revolution. Take it one step further and read about Himalayan Sea Salt. Reported to have 84 trace minerals contained in its crystals, it's just one more step in creating a perfectly healthy environment inside your body.

84 easily assimilated minerals- read more at www.himalayancrystalsalt.com .

Then there's yeast problem. Yeast is also known as candida or thrush.

When I was first diagnosed the healthcare professional would check me for thrush. I have since learned that yeast can destroy our health and harbor disease. It makes it difficult for us to lose weight and it thrives on our sugar intake, often surviving the antibiotics we abuse, and ruining healthy outcomes. I have found that probiotics are very helpful. Another item that physicians seem oblivious to.

High doses of probiotics will aid digestion, help clean out the intestines, and fight yeast. The same qualities can be found in fresh fruits and vegetables. I suggest eating better and using probiotics when needed. Foods first, always try to eat better as the main disease-fighting tactic.

Herbs and spices stimulate internal systems to work their best and probiotics (not grocery store types) as needed. Yes, yogurt is good. But medicinal doses of probiotics are different, and come in the billions! I recommend that you read about probiotics.

Claims of mushrooms fighting cancer may or may not be true, but I like the odds, and I love homemade mushroom soup- so I make homemade mushroom soup often.

I make homemade soup often! Most of what I eat is either raw or homemade- which that brings to mind microwaves.

Get rid of your microwave. Your food loses all nutritional value once it goes through a microwave. If your food has no nutritional value, why eat it? And seriously, very little micro-waved food even tastes good!

Microwave popcorn is disgusting!

Try popping it fresh in coconut oil. The popcorn pops up so delightful and perfect- no butter is needed to enjoy it. Add real butter and some quality salt and no microwave popcorn can compare!

HIV is a virus. It will attack your body and try to wear you down. Once it wears you down, other diseases are fatal to you. You must keep your body strong and not let it win. Yes, there is a stigma. There shouldn't be, but there is. It's not a disease that is easy to catch, you don't get it from kissing or sneezing or sharing a glass. You don't get AIDS, you get HIV and it ravages your body and your ability to heal leading to AIDS.

But I am healing just fine and my body is still fighting the virus. Maybe if we asked the people living 30 years with the virus what they do, or the Elite Controllers and Non Progressors what they do in their homemade alternative therapies we could get a better sense of what works and why. As long as there is no conversation about the people fighting the disease alone and in secret, we are wasting time and probably a lot of lives.

Someday they might realize that so many died needlessly due to lack of nutritional therapy and poor lifestyle choices. It will be a black mark on the medical community. It's not much different for cancer, diabetes, and many other debilitating conditions. Lifestyle and nutrition plan an important part. We are hurting ourselves. Don't abuse yourself and expect miracles from the medical establishment.

The doctors never ask if you're spraying pesticides all over the house or how many toxic food additives you consume on a daily basis. They will prescribe you a pill, or two or three, and then you have more chemicals in your already chemical laden life.

Eat to live. Eat simply and eliminate toxins from as much of your life as you can. Ask questions and find answers. Don't just settle for what you're told....we are all different and we can be amazing

Find healthy foods you like and consume them. I love potato chips but they aren't going to fight my viral load and stop it from replicating.

I am not fond of Turmeric or Curry, but Cauliflower Soup with Turmeric is a disease-fighting bowl of better health.

Foods to be eaten regularly should include a variety of colors, flavors, and textures. Consume many fresh fruits, vegetables, herbs, and spices.

Here is a list of some of the best foods to be eating regularly. Sure there's some you won't like, so don't eat them.

- Garlic
- Cayenne / Red Pepper
- Onion
- Turmeric
- Mushrooms
- Curry
- Celery
- Cumin
- Spinach
- Anise
- Kale, dark greens-all kinds
- Basil
- Leeks
- Oregano
- Cabbage
- Coriander
- Brussel sprouts
- Ginseng
- Parsley
- Honey
- Kim Chi
- Coconut, coconut oil, coconut flour, coconut cream, coconut milk

- Blackberries, raspberries, cherries, watermelon, strawberries, mulberries, blueberries
- Almonds, walnuts, pecans, cashews
- Cloves, nutmeg, and cinnamon
- Healthy grains- Quinoa, Bulgur Wheat, beans, and oatmeal
- Watermelon
- Kiwi
- Currants

It's important for you to read about the things I discuss in this book. There is an excellent book about the lymphatic system by Paul Chhabra titled *Healthy Self*. It doesn't try to sell you anything; it recommends ingredients available at the grocery store or in your garden. This isn't rocket science.

There are often disclaimers and warnings are posted about supplements and such things regarding HIV self-treatment. Sure, there are some supplements you could use, but caution is recommended when pharmaceuticals are already prescribed.

However, if you're newly diagnosed and not on medicines of any kind you have more options. You can start with pesto made with basil and move along to basil oil if you have no allergic reaction.

I'll soon be trying oregano oil. I hate oregano but it kills viruses! HIV is a virus so it makes perfect sense to me

A person I've chatted with claims a shot made of olive oil, cayenne, lemon, and garlic is a helpful tool. It makes sense olive oil helps clean you out and moisturizes, cayenne produces a sweat, garlic has sulfur and is alkaline, and lemon is also alkaline with vitamin C. Another person who has been HIV positive for 30 years recommends sweats as a medicinal healing tool. Increased circulation, something sick people rarely get is also very important. Who feels like a good, blood pumping, work out when you're miserable? But the increased blood circulation will help clean out sluggish lymph glands. Remember -the lymphatic system is where your immune system hides out. **A healthier lymphatic system = a healthier immune system.**

You have to decide what is important to you. A taste for cola products versus a taste for carrot juice, or any other healthy juice, is a personal choice. Whether you want white bread or nutritionally dense whole grain bread is up to you. You can cheat your health with microwaved garbage or learn to prepare and eat fresh wholesome foods that keep you younger, stronger, and healthier.

I remember watching beautiful young girls eat fast foods and garbage, and wonder where they got their energy. I am a very lethargic person, despite my raw food and healthy choices. Later I found out that cocaine and meth were the missing ingredients that gave those young girls so much energy. Now those beautiful young girls are hideous zombies if they are still alive. Many of them were much younger than I am and now look much older than I do.

When you start changing your food choices it can take months for the benefits to start to impact your health. So start ASAP! When you eat a bowl of berries, it takes a process for the berries benefits to reach your blood stream. Don't wait to change dietary habits. It only prolongs the miraculous benefits.

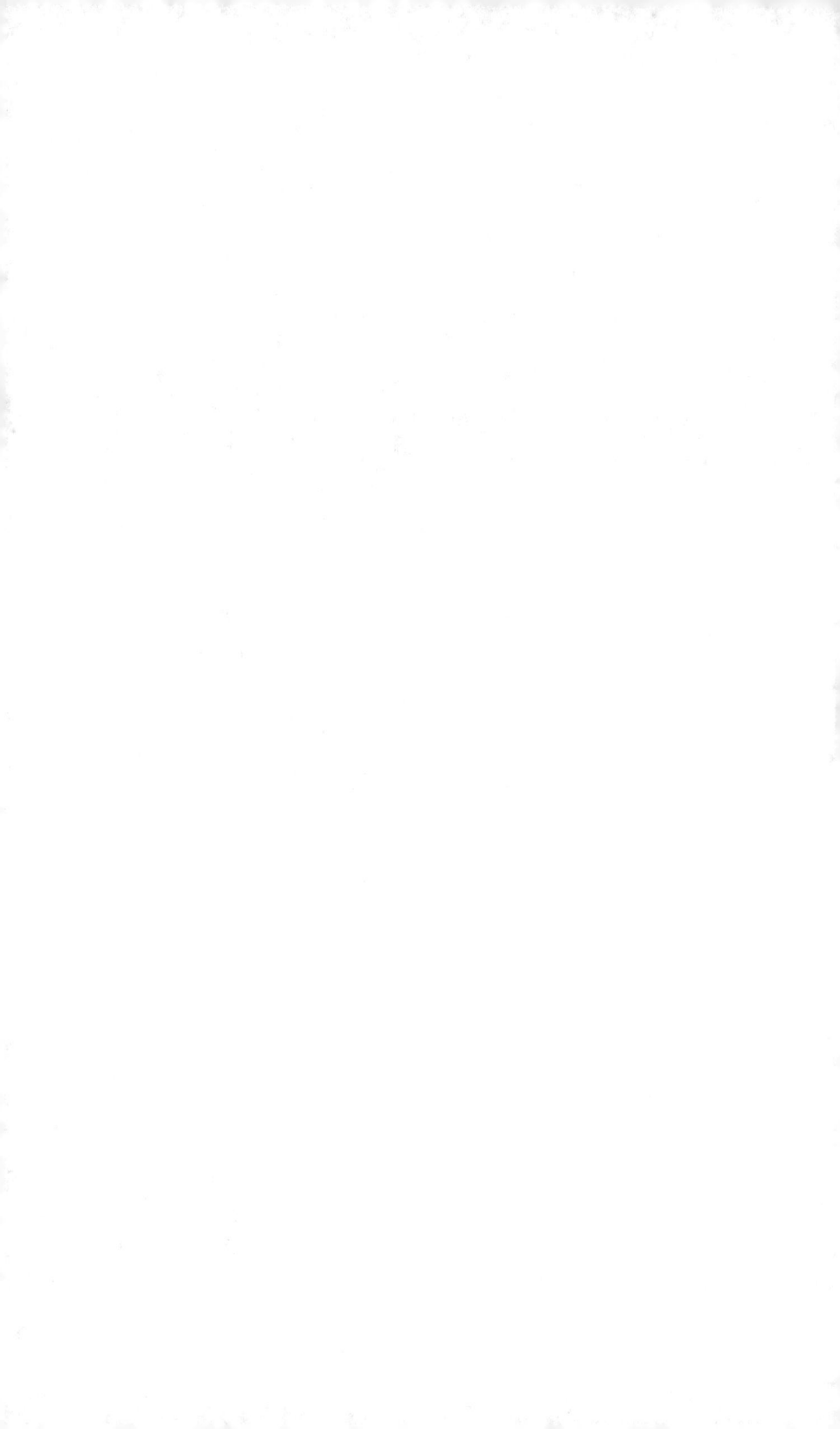

Soup Is Good For You

Most of what I eat is raw, unprocessed, and home cooked. I steam vegetables rather than boiling them in water. Salads are my main diet but soup can be a lymphatic system boost when you make it full of nutrient rich foods and aromatic spices.

Soup is the 'go to' food for health. It warms you and gives comfort and is often very nourishing, provided you make it yourself.

These are my favorite soups.

1. Onion Soup
2. Mushroom Soup
3. Onion Mushroom Soup
4. Potato Soup
5. Cabbage Soup
6. Tomato Soup
7. Cauliflower Soup
8. Split Pea Soup   (green, orange or yellow)
9. Bean Soup

I don't measure things out, just use what I need and flavor with what I have on hand.

Onion Soup /Onion and Mushroom Soup/ Mushroom Soup

Ingredients:

- A couple large onions or several small and medium ones
- Mushrooms for the mushroom version, raw or canned
- Soy sauce or beef broth
- Garlic if you choose
- PINK SALT
- Butter
- Depending on what version you choose
- Begin by sautéing the ingredients in butter.
- A light brown color change, and add water or broth.
- If using water, soy sauce adds excellent flavor, or try tamari….or a mushroom soup mix in a pinch…or an onion soup mix…(useful for a big pot of soup)

Instructions

If it's mushroom soup, then lots of mushrooms and a little onion.

If it's onion soup, then lots of onions and no mushrooms.

And if it's onion mushroom soup, be generous with both, enhancing your choice, the onions or the mushrooms!

Add pepper to taste, coarse black pepper if you like it, or white pepper for a kick

Potato Soup

Ingredients

- Large unblemished potatoes, of your favorite variety experiment or use what's on sale. White, Idaho, Reds, or Golden
- 1 stick of butter, or more for a big pot
- Onions -a little or a lot
- 1-2 cups milk (whole, ½, skim, or powdered)

Instructions

Wash potatoes or peel them if you want no skins

Slice up or cube or bigger pieces if cooking will be longer

Boil potatoes and onions in water, just enough to cover potatoes

Add ½ stick butter and salt and pepper to taste

When potatoes are tender add milk to make potato water creamy, it's really good with whole milk and some ½ and ½

Simmer on low, so the milk doesn't scald. only about 5 minutes

Serve with a slice of butter on top

May add cheese, bread crumbs, croutons, more onion, carrot or ham.

Cabbage Soup

Ingredients

- Depending on size of pot or kettle use ½ to 1 whole head of cabbage sliced and chopped roughly
- water
- 1 stick Butter
- Onions
- Carrots
- Tomatoes, canned or fresh, or tomato paste
- Some garlic, optional
- Rice, optional
- Chili powder or Cajun spice
- Cracked or crushed red pepper for the brave

Instructions

Sauté onions in butter in pot or kettle slightly

Add cabbage and water to almost cover the cabbage

Add tomatoes or tomato paste

Add carrots (optional)

Simmer

Depending on if you want rice or spice, add your choices

I once made it too spicy, and added a slight tablespoon of dark brown sugar to offset the heat…. it was yummy.

Tomato Soup

Ingredients
- Fresh or canned tomatoes
- Butter
- Spices you like
- Chili powder
- Cream, if you want creamy tomato

Instructions

Cook the tomatoes down

Remove the skins as the flesh falls off (compost the skins)

Add butter to taste, and spices or herbs of choice

Onions if you want

Garlic

Add cream at the end if that's your pleasure

A healthy grilled cheese makes a great companion to tomato soup.

I prefer no cream, and would add onion, garlic, and a squeeze of lemon at serving, or pour over noodles!

I remember my grandmother loved salty buttered noodles with canned tomatoes when she was sick.

Cauliflower Soup

This is an excellent source of turmeric.

Ingredients and Instructions

- Head of cauliflower broken into small pieces
- Steam it in water
- When nearly tender, add milk, or cream if calories are of no concern!

- ½ stick of butter
- ½ teaspoon of turmeric, more if you're accustomed to it
- Salt and pepper to taste

Pea Soup

There are several choices of split peas - orange, green, and yellow.

I prefer the orange and yellow split peas.

Simmer in water with ¼ stick of Butter and a small Onion

Add favorite spices or herbs- basil and chard are good choices.

This is good with a hearty slice of bread with butter

Bean Soup

Ingredients and Instructions
- Soak beans overnight. Rinse before using.
- Sauté onions in a soup pot.
- Add soaked Beans.
- Add a quart of water.
- Add garlic if you want.
- ½ stick of Butter

- You can add chili powder, Cajun spice mix, or diced tomatoes.
- Ham is another great addition if you want meat in your soup.
- Simmer on low, or prepare it in a crock pot, until beans are tender.
- Serve with a crusty bread and butter

Eliminating Toxins

Something few people talk about is elimination. It's a messy subject but it's possibly the most important factor in health. The garbage must come out! Daily bowel movements are critical to good health. Good circulation helps to remove the gunk from your system and deposit it into your waste removal process. Good health revolves around what you put in your body, via mouth, skin, and inhalation and then getting the waste products and toxins out.

This means that what you breathe or apply to your skin matters. What you do for a living can make a huge difference. Just ask about sickness among auto workers, nail techs, coal miners and so many others that work in toxic environments.

Take environmental factors into consideration too, and aim for a healthy environment. If HIV is attacking you inside and toxins are attacking you on the outside - it's an uneven battle. Good food is your tool to fight back. Sometimes you can't switch jobs but look for ways to protect yourself. Again, read about what affects you. My purpose is to say things others aren't and get you to be proactive about your health.

If I can fight the 'horrific HIV monster' with food and spices, what else is possible?

When you reach 50 your life is 1/2 over if you're planning to live to see 100! If you hope to see 70, you've lived 5/7's of your life by your 50th year. That is sad statistics. Waiting until you get to 50 years old to live healthy wasted precious years. Start today to make the effort to eat fresh and raw life-giving foods.

Older than 50? Get busy! Start juicing and drinking lemon and water. Use fresh lemons! Juicing delivers nutrients in the quickest and freshest form. Many believe juicing fights aging and disease. Just don't overdo juicing. It is critical that you also get fiber from the flesh and pulp of the fruits and vegetables. Juicing too much can provide too much of the sugars and not enough of the precious needed fiber.

The Best for Your Body

Alkaline Water

The body releases waste products, every cell has waste. It is acidic build-ups that may stimulate cancerous cells. Our bodies have a normal Ph. and an acidic or alkaline tendency. Sugars create an acidic Ph. Most vegetables are alkaline. Alkaline water claims to help remove acidic wastes better than water with a slight acidic Ph. i.e. normal tap water that is often fluoridated and chlorinated.

In a case of extreme healing and detoxifying, I'd say sure, get alkaline water; but a diet full of fruits and vegetables is also alkalinizing, so is lemon water.

I think quality salt is more important, and of course, water is water. The best water available is always nice, but not always a reality.

The Lymphatic System

While I was working on getting my Bachelor of Science in Health and Wellness one of the reference books, *Structure and Function*, opened my eyes to the limited information we get about the immune system.

Our immune system is in our lymphatic system. It is comprised of our spleen, thymus, red bone marrow, thoracic duct, tonsils, adenoids along with the lymph nodes and lymph vessels. Its defense function is BIOLOGICAL FILTRATION.

"The immune system is not simply a group of organs working together. Instead, it is a group of many organs and billions of freely-moving cells and trillions of free-floating molecules in many different areas of the body."

It's a moderately complicated process and to repeat it here for you would be plagiarism. I recommend a medical book, containing detailed information on the lymphatic system. It will help you understand CD4 and CD8 counts, T Cells, and the critical workings of the lymph glands and vessels. This is also critical information for cancer patients and those with other medical conditions. Understanding your lymphatic system will open up a big window into disease resistance. You will learn how being free of toxic and damaging substances will give you an important tool in remaining as healthy as you possibly can. If the first book you look at is too complicated or too simple, seek out others. It is your life, put some effort into it.

I recommended the book *Healthy Self* by Paul Chhabra. It has information from front to back on the inner workings of the lymphatic system, how to strengthen it, how to heal it, and how to drain it with massage and sweats.

Exercise is great for the immune system. Proper nutrition combined with exercise is crucial for a healthy lymphatic system. Paul Chhabra's background began with his grandmother and her traditional Indian (from India) healing practice. Herbs and spices play heavily in the technique, along with detoxification, dietary changes, and education and awareness. Most of his recommendations are free or inexpensive, readily available at the grocery store or in a garden. I bought his book for $5.00 on the internet.

Yeast, Thrush, and Chronic Yeast Infections

Do you have problems with yeast and thrush, are you are unable to lose weight or have chronic yeast infections? Slow healing?

Too much yeast in the body can cause flu-like symptoms. It can wreak havoc on the entire body. It thrives on sugar. Probiotics can help break it down. Doses of quality Probiotics in the billions will help digest food, break down intestinal build up, and destroy the yeast and bad bacteria. And unlike antibiotics, the probiotics will not destroy the good bacteria but will strengthen the good bacteria instead.

Brewer's Yeast

Brewer's Yeast is found in fermented foods. Examples include alcoholic beverages, aged cheeses, vinegar (an ingredient in salad dressings, ketchup, prepared mustard, mayonnaise, pickles, olives, steak sauce, barbecue sauce, etc.) Malt (an ingredient in many bowls of cereal and candies), soy sauce, cider, sauerkraut, and root beer. Brewer's Yeast is frequently used to fortify foods with B vitamins such as flour, bread, and cereals and is found in many nutritional supplements unless the label states "yeast free". These items should be avoided by individuals with Brewer's Yeast sensitivity. Some lower mold cheeses include the following: cottage cheese, cream cheese, ricotta, mozzarella, and Monterey Jack.

Baker's Yeast

Baker's Yeast is contained in yeast-leavened bread, rolls, buns, donuts, pastries, pizza dough, pretzels, some canned refrigerator biscuits, sourdough products, some crackers, some cookies, some canned soups, and some flour tortillas, etc. These foods should be avoided by individuals with Baker's Yeast sensitivity.

Malt

Malt is a product derived from barley or other grain. It is primarily used as a flavoring and coloring agent. It is a major ingredient of beer, ale, malt liquors, and non-alcoholic products like near beer and proprietary malt tonics. Most, though not all, dry breakfast cereals contain malt or malt extract as a flavoring agent. Crackers and Grape Nuts contain high quantities of malt.

Other foods that contain malt include: all baked goods, bread, pancake and waffle mix, biscuit mixes, cake mixes, soda crackers, confections, wheat flour, ice cream, candy, cake, baby cereal, malted milk, infant formulas, cooked breakfast cereal, dry breakfast cereal, potato chips, powdered milk, table syrup, malt extract, malt syrup, malt vinegar, soda fountain drinks, coffee substitutes, coffee and tea.

Natural Choices for the Eradication of Viruses

Here's a small list of some of the popular medicinal food sources and a brief explanation. I only want to peak your interest so you will read more on your own.

There are hundreds of Herbal books, home remedy books, and alternative healing books. You just need to start reading some of them for yourself. The information is out there, just not at the doctor's office.

Basil

Basil is readily available. You can grow your own or buy it at a farm stand. Homemade pesto will be much more effective than store bought options. Basil oil is pungent and a bit like anise in flavor. My viral load substantially dropped when I started using basil oil.

From The Healing Herbs: "Basil may also stimulate the immune system...One animal study showed basil stimulates the immune system by increasing production of disease-fighting antibodies by up to 20%."

Do not use basil when pregnant or nursing.

Oregano

Oregano is reported to be antiviral, anti-bacterial, and anti-microbial. It is easily found, easy to cook with, and easy to grow. Oregano oil could possibly wipe out most common illnesses and give the HIV virus a good stomping. I haven't used it yet, but I plan too.

Curry

Curry is not a common ingredient in American foods, but it makes many medicinal claims. Try it on cauliflower, in cauliflower soup, or on rice. It's an unusual flavor and may require some getting used to. The medicinal qualities may inspire you to try it. I encourage you to read more about it.

Turmeric

Turmeric has very little flavor and is often used to make Tofu yellow and to mimic eggs in the Vegan world. It also makes claims of better health when consumed regularly.

From the Healing Herbs: "Liver Protection: One study on animals showed curcumin has a protective effect on liver tissue exposed to liver-damaging drugs..."

Cayenne or Red Pepper

Cayenne, Jalapenos, and spicy foods rev up circulation and can sometimes get you to break into a sweat. Sweating is good! From The Healing Herbs: "The Red Pepper, or Capsicum, is used for Diabetic foot problems (by increasing circulation) and in severe Shingles cases."

Celery

Celery is a diuretic. It removes water from your body and is an excellent source of fiber and water. Celery Seed is also a good source of nutrients.

Mushrooms

Mushrooms are claimed to have anti-cancer compounds. Read about them. Different varieties offer different benefits.

Onions

Onions are very healthy. Read more about their benefits.

Garlic

Garlic is another germ and virus killer. If you don't eat onions, eat Garlic. If you don't like garlic…eat lots of onions.

Lemon, Lemon Oil

I have seen a drop of lemon oil dropped on Styrofoam, it melted a hole in it before my eyes, instantly. If it melts UN degradable Styrofoam, in theory, it will help to strip out the gunk from your cells. What gunk? The gunk from years of petroleum-based lotions, food chemicals, and plastic you've consumed via plastic dishes in the microwave.

Coconut Oil

Coconut Oil research claims that it can eat HIV virus. It has so many other health benefits as well, including lowering cholesterol, fighting Alzheimer's, heart health, and brain function. It may not cure HIV, but it's so good for you. You can cook with it, eat it with a spoon, or rub it on as a lotion. Try it as a lubricant; it is non-toxic and super slick.

Raw Honey

Although raw honey isn't recommended for babies under 2 years old, it's very good for a salve and sore throat. If your immune system is severely compromised, it would be better to use the pasteurized honey. But this book is about being healthy enough to have raw honey.

Consume Quinoa, Bulgur Wheat, Old-fashioned Oat Meal, Barley, Beans and Whole Grains for Protein and Fiber

Essential Oils

Essential Oils are a more complicated and intricate subject than the human body and all its systems (respiratory, lymphatic, digestive, skeletal, endocrine, muscular, nervous, urinary, and reproductive...).

Basil gives basil oil, sandalwood gives sandalwood oil, juniper- juniper oil, lemon-lemon oil, and so on.

These proprietary oils and essences have been thoroughly analyzed, revealing their chemical compounds in amazing detail. I can't begin to describe the 1000's of benefits and scientific reasons why. But there are books out there that do, and you'll be amazed.

Aromatherapy is an Essential Oils 'discipline', and most oils can be used for aromatic uses, but not all oils are consumable.

Some will be too strong to apply to the skin (Cinnamon for example) and some will be consumable, such as food grade frankincense.

You should learn the difference between perfume oils, medicinal oils, and pure essential oils. Some oils are food grade and edible or topical, while some are just cosmetic.

The cosmetic oils are not what we are looking for. Often the price is a factor, essential oils are an intense and expensive process with 3 tons of plant material yielding 1 pound of oil in some cases.

A good essential oil extraction process will not reach high enough temperatures to kill the very thing you are after (usually <180 degrees), the life force of the plant!

None of this is *mumbo jumbo*. Scientists, healers, and farmers have all studied most of what I have listed, and many, many more. Essential Oils have been broken down in laboratories to their very basic chemistry and ancient herbal methods have been confirmed by modern day science.

One of the best sources of pure essential oils, collected and extracted in the highest of quality, is **Young Living Essential Oils**. They surpass the standard, often growing and harvesting the desired material, and literally seeking to extract the living essences of the mother plant for the greatest benefits in the human body.

Essential Oils are highly concentrated. Some are able to pass thru the blood/ brain barrier connecting with you on a cellular level even when the vapors are inhaled, as in Aromatherapy.

Food grade, non-toxic consumable oils are the medicinal forms and this is very important! You can apply them to pulse points, add drops of them to bath water or consume in a glass of water or tea. Simple and painless.

My basil oil is in a roll on applicator, and I use it as lip gloss. Sometimes I rub it on pulse points (neck, wrist, behind knees). Why? It's anti-viral and absorbed through the skin. I apply it to the lymph nodes and vessel areas.

Read and Research

It is my hope you're still reading, and that I touched some topics you weren't aware of or had maybe wondered about. That I took away some of your fear and anxiety and helped you to understand why food is so important for optimal health and longevity. I merely scratched the surface and ask that you seek out additional reference sources and read expanded versions of my commentary and opinions. It's an ongoing experiment. I am my own lab rat.

Many of my reference books were obtained second hand at used bookstores, and of course, the internet has many sources. If hundreds of people make claims about the benefits of coconut oil and only a few disagree...I tend to listen to the hundreds.

When I read the immune system is a complicated process inside the lymphatic system it makes me mad as hell we don't get such information. It is very frustrating to try to open up a dialog with your doctor and only get unproductive information and no real answers.

Learn how to read your lab work. From CD4 and CD8 to your liver panel and cholesterol levels, to your white blood count and all the rest- understand what those numbers mean. Be proactive on your own behalf! You have so much to gain; it really is a matter of life and death.

So what do I do exactly? I drink a lot of coffee and I eat a lot of real butter. I am not perfect but I eat mostly fresh fruits and vegetables, whole wheat bread and real mayonnaise. I use coconut oil and sunflower oil. I eat eggs, cheese, and lots of homemade soup. Cabbage soup, onion and garlic soup, potato soup, and mushroom soup.

I don't take vitamins, but when I do I look for whole food sources, not chemical compounds replicated in a lab. I never use a microwave. I use basil oil on pulse points and as a lip gloss. I use a lot of and herbs and spices when I cook.

I could wait a few more years to write this book, a few more months and proofread it over and over again, add more detail... but the other books you need are already out there.

The herb books and natural healing books don't require re-writing, especially not by me.

I want to get this out so people can stop being so afraid and get tested, so people without health care can take better care of themselves, so HIV stops spreading and to open up a new conversation about what works.

I had to study this on my own, playing with food choices and lifestyle changes and I think it's time to share how healthy I am maintaining my levels.

Read the labels on your foods, stay away from items with more than 5 ingredients. Always avoid high fructose corn syrup and propylene glycol alginate.

Avoid environmental toxins as much as possible- bus fumes, chemicals, paint fumes, oven cleaner- all the stuff that requires ventilation.

Eat a variety of colorful foods and spices. Avoid micro-waved foods and choose foods that are closer to still being 'alive'- this means fresh fruits, vegetables, and herbs. Eat raw as much as possible. Avoid over processed and over cooked foods.

Let's sum things up-

Coconut Oil is a necessary part of a healthy lifestyle.

Basil oil and oregano oil kill viruses.

Food-based nutrition is crucial.

Exercise is important.

Sweating out toxins is necessary.

Essential Oils are not all created equal. You want food grade and edible oils. You need non-toxic oils, not perfume oil or topical/light bulb style oils. Young Living Essential Oils or Scentuallyyours.com is two excellent sources of oils. Those Nature People in Frankenmuth, Michigan are also an excellent resource.

Stress Kills

Laughter Heals

Read more, don't stop here. There are so many health books, herb books, and healing books out there.

I am beating HIV & AIDS with healthy lifestyle choices.

Don't give up and don't waste time killing yourself with junk food, soda pop, and chemicals and preservatives.

And don't condemn your kids to an early death, or a life of ill health feed them healthy from the start.

Reference Books

Reference Guide for Essential Oils by Connie and Alan Higley

The Healing Herbs, The Ultimate Guide to the Curative Power of Nature's Medicine by Michael Castleman

Structure and Function of the Body 13th Edition by Thibodeau and Patton   Prepared by Linda Swisher

Healthy Self by Paul Chhabra

Modern Encyclopedia of Herbs by Joseph Maidens, N.D. Ph.D.

Herbally Yours by Penny C. Royal

Neal's Yard Natural Remedies by Susan Curtis, Romy Fraser & Irene Kohler

The Complete Book of Incense, Oils, and Brews by Scott Cunningham

Links and Reference Sources

HIV-related

www.zephyrfoundation.org

www.thetribe.com

www.agirllikeme.org

Essential Oils

www.YoungLiving.com

www.AbundantHealth4u.com

www.globalscents.com

www.http://scentuallyyours.com

Herbs and Spices and Alternative Healing information

www.thosenaturepeople.com

Brands and Specific Types

Tropical Traditions Coconut Oil

Pink Himalayan Crystal Salt

A   Comprehensive list of Toxins in our Food and Beauty Care Products can be found at:

www.LivingAnointed.com

Best Wishes for Your Good Health

Of course, you could just take the medicine…but you should also eat better to keep your body as strong as possible.

Fighting disease isn't easy, and the best way to think about it is like an animal breeder. A breeder invests his money on the health of his animal and good feed is often the number one investment. Why would we care more for livestock diets than we do our own or our children's'?

For genetic strength, for disease resistance, for a strong immune system, the key is to eat healthier.

Labs, Alternative Meds, and General Observations

My diagnosis came in January 2005. Here are a series of lab results.

	2005 March/July/ November	2006 APRIL	2007 March/June Nov. wasp attack
Viral Load	/113/75	135	689/3304/ 4042/24967
CD4	584/765/625	553	528/566/624
CD8	370		292/411
HDL			/56
LDL			93/92
Triglyceride			58/74
CHOLESTEROL			168/163
WBC			5.6/4.9
RBC			4.67/4.71

	2008	2009	2010
	JUNE	January	January
Viral Load	1654		1979/873
CD4	560		472/625
CD8			637/697
HDL			67
LDL			106
Cholesterol			184
Triglycerides			54

	2011 January	2012 January	2013 January
Viral Load	1849		290
CD4	677		345
CD8	667		445
HDL	65		67.
LDL	105		95.
Cholesterol	188		176
Triglycerides	89		
WBC	5.		4.32
RBC	4.63		4.40
			.

June 2013

8 years after my original diagnosis they have a new formula for the criteria for meds. Because my CD4's were low, the conversation turns to the pharmaceuticals. Totally bypassing the 209 Viral Load, but there was no conversation about that.

I could be wrong, but what if I am right? Or just onto something?

After I got stung by a bunch of wasps, my viral load hit upwards of 20,000. I was devastated. This was my time to start replicating the virus obviously. Well, the next Labs showed it in the 1000's, not 40,000's like I expected.

Then the viral load went down to 290 with no prescription meds, no modern medical interference. No comments from the doctors.

If the viral load starts to increase again I'll become even more dedicated to healthy food therapy.

Currently, it's 2017 and I am fine.

I have had some ups and downs, and my CD 4 has too. I even went into AIDS status with a 195 CD4, but I eliminated the thing that was causing me great stress and my numbers jumped back up to the high 600's. Pretty amazing, huh?

I wish I could tell you more specific things, some golden bit of info that would help everyone, but it's a compendium of healthy stuff. Good health is cumulative.

I have not made it to a steam room, yet. I had planned on monthly sweats to both revs up the immune (Lymphatic) system and lose weight but that hasn't happened. It is still on my to-do list though.

I have tried colloidal silver and have continued using basil oil, clove oil, and any other essential oils I could afford. I consume cinnamon regularly in my coffee or as cinnamon tea. I use coconut oil often, though I never did eat spoonfuls of it. Coconut cream yes, coconut oil- No. But it does make nice lip balm.

I opt for the greenest veggies, the richest oranges in carrots, and lots of beets. I have taken charcoal tablets to pull out toxins, and chlorella supplements for added nutrition. Herbs and spices are your best friends, consume what you love and can tolerate.

I eat a ton of garlic and onion sandwiches, I am still a vegetarian.

If you're not a vegetarian I recommend high-quality meats.

If you think you're not worth it, think again. Don't sell yours or your kids' health short; good nutrition does make a difference.

More about the stressful event put me into AIDS.

I wasn't worried or surprised; I knew the *Jerry Springerish* things going on in my life were going to bottom me out. So many tears, so much anger, confusion, and stress. As soon as I took a deep breath and began the process of removing myself from the drama, my levels got right back to where they should be. Even I was amazed. But the Doctors I don't think they don't give a damn. They seem to be disengaged, oblivious, stymied, or maybe completely befuddled. I don't know what to call it, but it's of no damn help to me at all.

But my levels are perfect! And I strive for undetectable or better!

And I did this with no modern medicine. Only alternative therapies and healthy foods.

Is it too much work? I don't think it's too much work to stay healthy and alive. I do know I wouldn't adhere to the meds. I am terrible at routine, I hate going to the doctor's office- especially after this fiasco. I have no trust in the doctors their minds are not open to the possibilities beyond their prescription pad.

I can't afford an alternative medical practitioner plus they are pretty rare in Flint, Michigan. Yes, that Flint, Michigan. With the water crisis.

I never quit using the water. My coffee is perked on the stove and I eat plenty of green leafy veggies so my lead level is only 4. Flint is an industrial town and we have bad water. A 4 is good.

I can't give any "expert medical advice" only anecdotal observations and stories about what has worked for me. I am an HIV positive patient on a mission to live and not succumb to ignorance or experimentation by someone else. I know food heals; it is what the human body requires to sustain health and beat invaders like the flu, HIV, and the common cold.

It's liberating to not need twelve or more pharmaceuticals to survive on a daily basis. Not referring to just HIV medicines either. So many people, even those younger than me, take so many prescriptions. Other than HIV I also have no other health issues. No high blood sugar or Diabetes, no high blood pressure, and no sleeping problems (though I do sleep too much). I don't have any of the other *pick your poison* 'maladies' the medical community can put a name on and write a prescription for.

If you feel your health isn't worth the effort, the money, or the care needed to beat the system at its own game, then maybe could you at least care for your kids' health (if you have them) and see the difference proper nutrition can make.

A Thank You from the Author

Thank you for your interest, and your indulgence. Your health is your choice, you can make up for lost time wasted, but don't wait any longer. Value your children's health, even before conception, by taking care of yourself. Why should animal breeders guard their bloodlines health and genetics better than we humans do? Whether it's a horse breeder, a pedigree dog breeder, or a 4H rabbit or goat breeder they put in what they hope to get out!

YOU ARE WHAT YOU EAT

And one last bit of advice- play lots of whatever music you love to listen to.

Play music whenever you're feeling sorry for yourself, when you are afraid of what's ahead, or when you are lonely! Be good to yourself. Eat to Live!

Thank You,

~ S. Diane Barry